WHY AM I NOT LOSING WEIGHT?

Discover the Secrets to Effective and Sustainable Weight Loss

Dr. Pietro C. Alvero

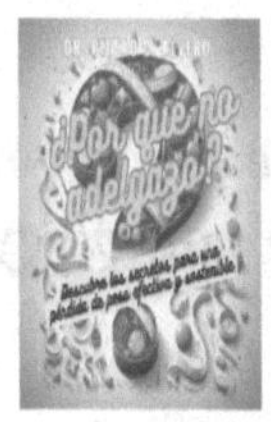

"Obstacles don't have to stop you. If you run into a wall, don't turn around and give up. Figure out how to climb it, go through it, or work around it."

Michael Jordan

To Ana Belén, for helping me put into practice,
by getting my hands dirty, all the theory and
science of the fascinating world of sports.

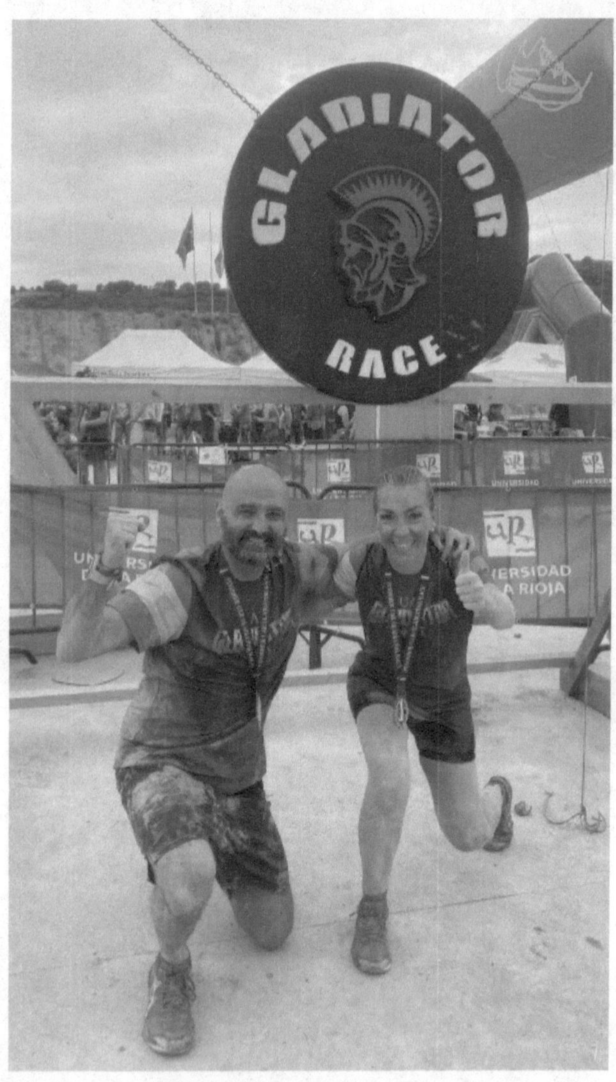

Author's Note

Why Am I Not Losing Weight?

Dear reader, if you are reading these pages, it is because, surely, after having tried many diets, you are still asking yourself the same question... Why on earth am I not losing weight?

If you think that in this book you will find a new miracle diet to help you shed those stubborn pounds in a few days, I'm sorry to say that you might as well close it (or turn it off, if it's an e-book) and dive into a science fiction novel where, in the end the same thing will happen as if you were to embark on another fantastic diet that promises you the world. If, on the other hand, you trust in yourself, in the physiology of your body, in the strength of your mind, and, why not say it, in new technologies, then you can keep reading, as I hope that the following pages will help you achieve our shared goal.

Before deciding to write this book, I had already treated many patients who came to my practice with that same question. Almost all of them, with few exceptions, asked me the same thing (which is why this book has its title) and claimed to have followed hundreds of miracle diets that promised the moon and the stars without achieving any positive results. I will not waste a second of our valuable time describing any of the most famous ones, but it is true that, while some may indeed reduce a certain percentage of body mass, it is no less true that the vast majority end up affecting health and, after a short time, returning you to your original weight, in the best of cases.

As you will come to understand while reading these pages, losing weight is not something impossible; quite the opposite. However, it requires more than just eating proteins, eliminating all carbohydrates, or fasting for half the day. The latter, fasting, is something I can partially affirm works. It is a good measure as long as other factors are taken into account, which I will explain in more detail in the coming chapters. However, it should never be done without any control, and even less so should you believe that during the allowed eating period, you can raid the fridge as if there were no tomorrow.

You will observe, page by page, that the book is written in a relaxed tone with the aim of making you feel as comfortable as possible and paying attention to everything detailed in it. However, you should not forget its rigor, and, as it cannot be otherwise, that it is based on the empirical results that any scientific work requires, no matter how accessible and simple the reading may be. I could have chosen to write a guide with the same content as the book you have in your hands, using complicated medical terminology under the pretext of giving it greater scientific pomp, but that is not precisely what I believe the reader is looking for. As you will see, I have omitted all medical jargon and, at least I believe, its content is completely accessible to any reader, regardless of their medical knowledge. In fact, I haven't needed to include a single explanatory footnote, as, although I do mention some medical terms, they are all known by the vast majority of the population.

Finally, all that remains is to hope that this book meets your expectations. Keep one thing in mind: the book itself... will not make you lose weight! You could try putting it on the barbecue, as the calories in the paper are almost zero, but I don't think its taste will be particularly pleasant (I don't even want to think about the e-book) but seriously, as we move through its chapters and you start to absorb its key points (which I will repeat continuously) you will realize that if you put fifty percent of its content into action, you will at least be able to answer the initial question. And when you know the solution to a problem, it is much easier to solve it.

Don't wait any longer, put down that bag of snacks you have in your hands, and join the many people who have managed to shed those extra pounds, so that soon you can ask yourself... *Why on earth wasn't I losing weight?*

Then... Why am I not losing weight?

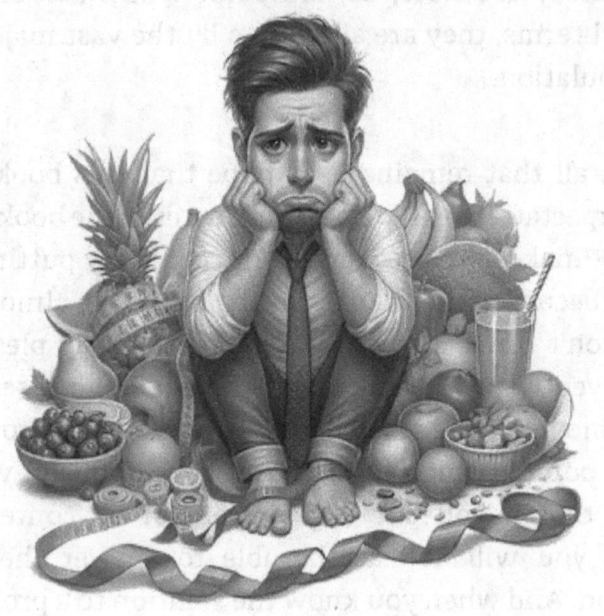

So... why am I not losing weight?

Losing weight can be a real challenge, and often we find ourselves wondering why we can't shed those extra pounds. To begin with, magic diets that promise quick results are a trap. Skipping meals, eliminating entire food groups, or following extreme diets may work for a while, but they are unsustainable in the long run and often leave us feeling hungrier and more frustrated.

Next, there's the somewhat taboo topic that is essential: exercise. We all know we need to move, but finding the motivation to do so is another story. It's not about killing yourself at the gym every day; it's about finding a routine that you genuinely enjoy and can maintain. Exercise should be something you naturally incorporate into your life in a pleasant way.

Psychology also plays a crucial role in this battle. Stress, anxiety, boredom, and other emotions can lead us to overeat. Additionally, being too self-critical can demotivate us and make us abandon our efforts before seeing results.

Another common issue is having unrealistic expectations. We want immediate results, but healthy weight loss takes time. Patience and consistency are essential, even though it can be challenging to maintain them at times.

We live in the digital age, and sedentary behavior is a constant threat.

Between office work, marathon TV series sessions, and endless scrolling on social media (where we mindlessly move our screens around) we spend a lot of time sitting. Less movement means fewer calories burned, which makes weight loss more challenging. Mindless eating is another silent enemy. Eating in front of the TV, snacking between meals, and giving in to late-night cravings can add up to many extra calories without us realizing it. Being aware of our eating habits is essential for managing calorie intake.

Lastly, biological factors such as genetics, metabolism, and hormones can also work against us. While not an excuse, these factors should be considered when developing appropriate and realistic strategies. In this case, the guidance of a specialist doctor can be crucial to the success of our approach. Even with the help of artificial intelligence, blindly relying on apps or devices without understanding how they work or without adapting them to your specific needs can lead to frustration. Technology can be a useful tool, but it cannot do all the work for you.

Losing weight, therefore, is not just about willpower but about understanding your body and mind, and adopting a balanced and sustainable approach. The key is patience and consistency. Within these pages, you will find advice and tools to finally and enjoyably lose weight and keep it off for good.

1. Obesity, a global health problem

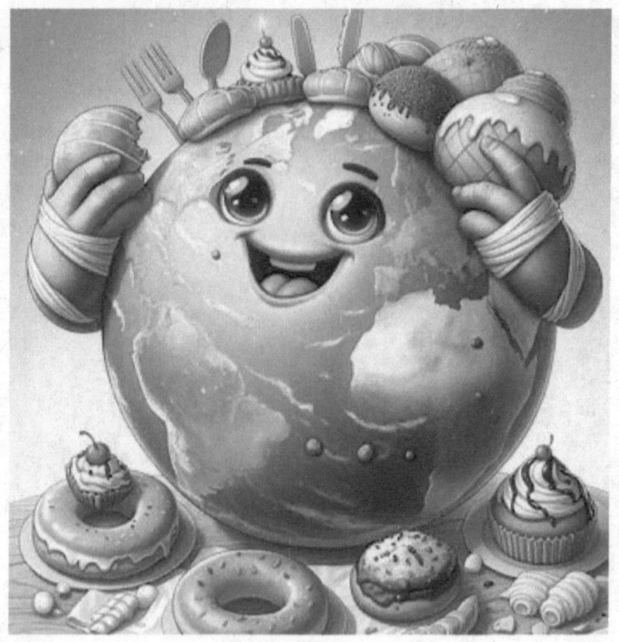

O besity, a Global Health Issue

Obesity and overweight have become critical issues in today's society, affecting millions of people worldwide. These problems not only impact physical appearance but are also associated with a range of serious diseases such as type 2 diabetes, heart disease, hypertension, and certain types of cancer. The rise in obesity rates is due to a combination of factors, including easy access to highly caloric and nutritionally poor foods, sedentary lifestyles, and a culture that promotes excessive consumption and convenience over physical activity. Additionally, advertising and the availability of fast and processed food have exacerbated this situation.

The economic and social costs of obesity are enormous. Healthcare systems are increasingly strained by the need to treat weight-related diseases, and affected individuals often face stigma and self-esteem issues. What is clear is that obesity and overweight pose significant challenges for public health, requiring comprehensive approaches that include education, health policies, and lifestyle changes to reverse this alarming trend.

But... what is the solution to achieve effective results?

Addressing the issue of overweight and obesity from multiple perspectives is crucial for achieving effective and lasting results. It's not just about counting calories or exercising, but about understanding and addressing a variety of factors that contribute to this complex problem, and that is one of the goals of this book.

From a nutritional perspective, it is essential to promote a balanced diet that not only aids in weight loss but also improves overall health. Regarding exercise, it is vital to find physical activities that are sustainable and enjoyable, tailored to individual needs. Psychology also plays a significant role, as emotional factors such as stress, anxiety, and depression can influence eating habits and motivation for exercise. Understanding and managing these emotions is fundamental for long-term success.

Furthermore, considering biological factors such as genetics and metabolism allows for the development of personalized and realistic strategies. Technology, as we have discussed, including artificial intelligence, can provide valuable tools for monitoring progress and customizing weight loss plans.

2. Nutrition, that great un-KNOWN

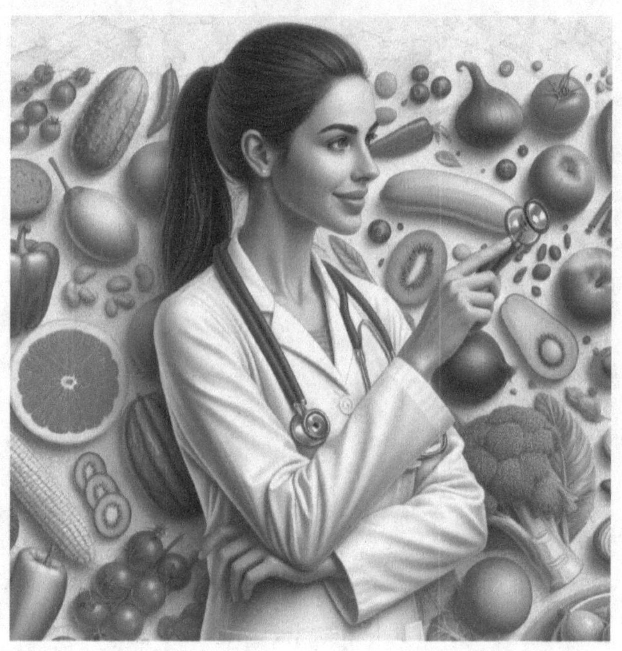

Fundamentals of a Healthy Diet

I don't intend, at this point, to explain what makes us gain weight, what agrees with us, or which foods we should avoid overindulging in. On these topics, everything has been written and analyzed extensively; however, the challenge, and why you are reading this book, lies in putting this knowledge into practice. Rather than delving into the scientific and medical physiology of nutrition in the human metabolism, I aim to break down, briefly and simply, the main challenges we face when we approach the refrigerator. Eating healthily doesn't have to be a headache. In fact, the fundamentals of a healthy diet are quite straightforward, and with a bit of common sense, anyone can follow them.

First and foremost, forget right now about fad diets that eliminate entire food groups. Your body needs a bit of everything: proteins, carbohydrates, healthy fats, vitamins, and minerals. The miracle diet does not exist! Once we grasp this principle, we will have started our weight loss journey on the right foot. Popular wisdom already establishes the solution for weight loss: *"less on the plate and more on the shoe."*

Repeat after me: *The miracle diet does not exist! The miracle diet does not exist!*

Repeat it until your brain gets it clear. Once you've internalized that *mantra,* you can continue reading. Are you clear now? Have you stopped believing in the miracle of the high-protein diet, the lipid diet, or the infamous *chicken-pineapple diet?* Well then, now you can continue...

Imagine your plate as a rainbow. The more natural colors it has (no, not those from bakeries) the better. Vegetables and fruits of all colors provide different nutrients that your body will appreciate. And speaking of appreciation, your heart and waistline will greatly thank you if you avoid, or rather, rationalize, ultra-processed foods and sugary drinks. Opt for fresh and natural foods whenever possible. You can also choose zero-calorie drinks, but make sure these beverages are truly zero (or close to zero) calories. Stay away from products that loudly advertise *"0% added sugars and/or fats."* What do you mean, *added?* Zero means zero, here and everywhere else, and if the label says *"added,"* it means they already added too many, and all they're limiting is adding even more... *quite clever*, as they say in my hometown.

Portion sizes matter too. Eating healthy doesn't mean you can indulge in a mountain of anything healthy. Remember, cows only eat grass... Controlling portions is key to not overloading your system. And above all, don't forget to stay hydrated. Water is your best friend on this journey. Drink plenty; after all, a full stomach, even if it's with liquid, is a stomach that has less room for food. Before each meal, drink two glasses of water. After five minutes, you can sit down to enjoy your lunch, and you'll find yourself feeling satisfied soon.

Pro Tip*:* To avoid becoming a water addict (a person with an impulsive desire to drink large amounts of water without being thirsty) you can alternate water intake with other low-calorie liquids such as teas, black coffees (you can add sweeteners, but avoid sugar), or even zero-calorie sodas.

Consider that caffeine or theine are stimulants that increase metabolic consumption without providing any calories, so hydrating with these types of beverages can be very beneficial for our weight loss project. Always with relative caution, as the sodium content of these drinks should always be considered.

And one more thing, say goodbye to the so-called energy drinks, which not only provide large amounts of carbohydrates but also pose a significant health risk. Certainly, the consumption of coffee or tea is contingent upon the individual having good blood pressure levels, as these beverages are contraindicated in cases of hypertension. In such instances, individuals can opt for decaffeinated varieties in moderation. For those with obesity or significant overweight, which often coexist with high blood pressure, alternating with flavored waters or caffeine-free herbal teas is advisable. It's important to note that in a high percentage of people (with the exception of congenital hypertension or pre-existing conditions) obesity and high blood pressure are associated, meaning weight loss can help improve vascular pressure levels.

Myths and Truths About Weight Loss Diets

Who hasn't heard the miraculous promise of losing 10 kilograms (22 lbs) in a week? Let's unravel some of the most common myths and set the record straight!

Here are seven of the most recurrent myths that we've all heard or read about weight loss. Behind these myths, there's obviously a hidden truth. A truth that everyone should know before embarking on the journey to achieve a healthy weight.

<u>Myths</u>

Myth 1: "Don't Eat Carbohydrates If You Want To Lose Weight!"

Carbohydrates are not your mortal enemies. Obviously, if you gobble down a loaf of bread every day, it won't help your waistline. But whole carbohydrates, like oatmeal, brown rice, and fruits, are important sources of energy and fiber. You just need to eat them in moderation and wisely. Another thing to note: whole grains can also contribute to weight gain. This doesn't mean that whole carbohydrates are less healthy than refined ones, but we must remember that whole doesn't equate to zero calories.

Myth 2: "Fat Makes You Fat."

Not all fats are bad. Healthy fats, such as those found in avocado, nuts, and olive oil, are essential for your body. They can even help you feel full and satisfied, preventing snacking binges.

Myth 3: "Skipping Meals Is A Good Way To Reduce Calories."

Skipping meals can slow down your metabolism and make you so hungry that you end up eating everything in sight.

It's better to eat regularly and in controlled portions.

Myth 4: "Only Strict Diets Work."

Super strict diets may give you quick results, but they are hard to sustain, and often the weight returns once you stop the diet. It's more effective to adopt healthy habits for the long term.

Myth 5: "Diet And Sugar-Free Products Are The Key."

Many "*diet*" or "*sugar-free*" products contain other ingredients that may not be good for you, such as artificial sweeteners and sodium. Additionally, marketing strategies often distort the message with claims like *"0% added sugars"* leading consumers to believe they are *calorie-free*. They can also give you a false sense of security and make you eat more than necessary.

Myth 6: "If You Exercise A Lot, You Can Eat Whatever You Want."

While exercise is important, you can't compensate for a poor diet with extra hours in the gym. The key is to find a balance between diet and exercise.

Myth 7: "Drinking Cold Water Burns More Calories."

It's true that your body uses a bit of energy to heat cold water to body temperature, but it's not enough to make a significant difference in your weight loss. It's preferable to end your daily shower with a good, refreshing blast of cold water. This can help wake you up for the day ahead and slightly increase calorie expenditure as your body returns to its optimal 98.6°F (37°C) temperature for proper function.

H ad you heard them before, right?

What should be clear to us, after analyzing this chapter, is that losing weight in a healthy way has no hidden secrets or magical shortcuts. It's a matter of balance, eating a bit of everything, and being consistent.

So, the next time you hear a promise of a miracle diet, remember: if it sounds too good to be true, it probably is.

Nutritional Decalogue for Sustainable Weight Loss.

Let's get straight to the point!

It's time to put it in black and white and present the main decalogue you should follow to improve your diet and lose weight sustainably, all without driving yourself crazy in the process. It may seem obvious, but implementing this will immediately impact your weight and physical fitness.

So, take out your phone and snap a picture of the following decalogue so you can carry it with you everywhere. In a few days, you won't need to review this list again because you'll have incorporated it into your daily routine. But initially, as simple as it may seem, it's important to have it handy to glance at quickly from time to time. Don't worry, soon it will become second nature.

The Decalogue of Healthy Weight Loss

1. Eat Slower

Did you know that it takes your brain about 20 minutes to register that you're full? Eating slowly helps your nervous system realize when you're satisfied, so chew well and enjoy every bite.

2. Don´T Skip Meals

Skipping breakfast will make you arrive at the next meal feeling ravenous, leading to overeating. Similarly, both mid-morning snacks -avoid sweets, though- and afternoon snacks are important. If you have to skip one of the five meals, let it always be dinner. Keep in mind that when you sleep, you're not hungry. In short, eat regularly to keep your metabolism running and avoid binges.

3. Fill Your Plate With Colors

No, we're not talking about *Haribo gummy bears* (you've read it in the advert voice, and you know it). Fill your plate with a rich variety of fruits and vegetables. The more colors, the more nutrients. Plus, it makes your meals much more appealing.

4. Plan Your Meals

Planning is key. Dedicate some time each week to plan your meals and grocery shopping. This way, you'll avoid resorting to fast food and impulsive decisions when hunger strikes. And never go grocery shopping when you're hungry.

5. Drink More Water

Water is essential, and sometimes we confuse thirst with hunger. Always carry a bottle with you, whether it's plain water or flavored water or other infusions, and make sure to drink enough throughout the day. Plus, water has zero calories, so it's your perfect ally.

Pro Tip: Drink two glasses of water before your main meals - breakfast and lunch - and one before dinner. Among other reasons, if you drink two or more glasses before dinner, you'll remember me every time you have to get up to go to the bathroom. You'll notice how it helps you feel fuller sooner.

6. Control Your Portions

Often it's not just about what you eat, but how much you eat. Use smaller plates to control portions and avoid overeating without realizing it. It may sound silly, but it will help your brain process that the amount is adequate for its needs.

7. Don´T Forbid Yourself Anything

Prohibiting certain foods will only make you crave them more. Instead, enjoy your indulgences in moderation. A piece of dark chocolate won't ruin your diet, but eating a whole bar every day might. You can also substitute them with *low-calorie* bars or snacks. These supplements are not magical, but they definitely provide fewer calories than a regular chocolate bar.

8. Get Enough Sleep

Sleep is crucial for your overall well-being and weight control. Lack of sleep can increase your appetite and make you seek out high-calorie foods to stay awake. Plus, did you know that calories are also burned while sleeping?

9. Cook At Home

Cooking your own meals allows you to control what you eat and how it's prepared. Experiment with healthy recipes and make cooking a fun activity.

Pro Tip 1: Try drinking one or two glasses of water (or cold infusions) while cooking. This will help you arrive at mealtime feeling less hungry, maintain hydration, and boost metabolism.

Pro Tip 2: If you're someone who enjoys spicy food, go for it. Spiciness is a great metabolism booster and increases body temperature, leading to energy expenditure. Of course, use caution or your stomach might protest.

10. Do Not Obsess Over The Scale

Weight fluctuates for many reasons, so don't obsessively weigh yourself every day. Focus on how you feel and the positive changes in your habits and energy levels. Weighing yourself once a week is sufficient for maintaining good weight control. And remember to do it always at the same time of day, preferably in the morning and before breakfast.

As you may have noticed, these ten points are easy to incorporate into your daily life and do not require drastic changes. It's simply about making small adjustments that, one by one, lead to significant long-term results.

Despite everything discussed in this chapter, we should never forget the crucial role played by our Primary Care Physician. They should be the ones to monitor your progress and, if they deem it necessary and your weight loss exceeds BMI thresholds, they can also assist with pharmacotherapy. Currently, there are several medications, approved by most national health agencies, that can greatly aid in weight loss for those facing serious health issues. When combined with other medical therapies such as mesotherapy or other cost-effective medical-aesthetic techniques available today, the results can be remarkable. However, I emphasize that these specific treatments should be prescribed by our Primary Care Physician or a specialist.

So, go ahead and take charge!

3. Exercise, a crucial factor...
But not the only one.

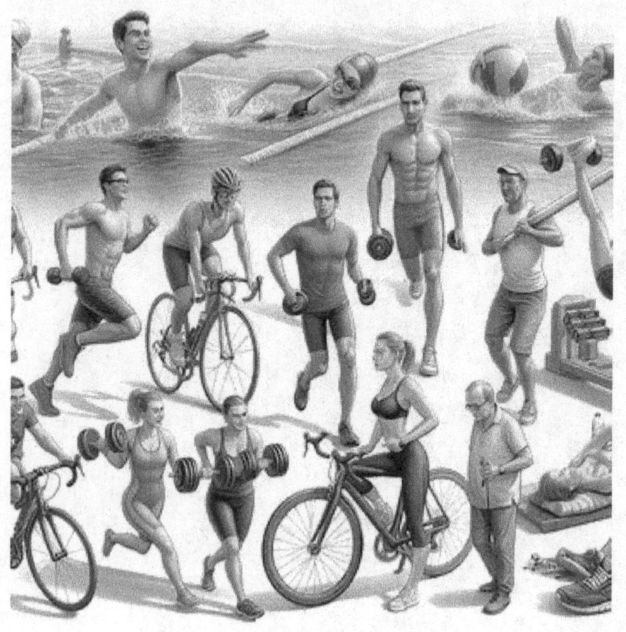

Exercise, a factor that is more than essential... but not the only one.

It's clear by now that nutrition is one of the main pillars of your weight loss project. However, as you might have suspected, the plan will be incomplete without adding regular physical exercise. Exercise doesn't necessarily have to be high-intensity, but it should be consistent. If you want to lose weight in a healthy way and, above all, maintain it, physical exercise is your best ally.

Here, I'll explain to you in an illustrative way why movement is crucial.

Physical and Mental Benefits of Exercise

Calorie Burning

Firstly, exercise helps burn those extra calories you consume. Imagine your body is like a bank account: if you deposit more calories than you spend, you accumulate a "balance" (in the form of fat). Moving more helps you expend those calories and reduce the accumulated balance. So, how about giving your calorie account a break?

Boosts Your Metabolism

Exercise, especially strength training like lifting weights or doing squats, increases your muscle mass. Muscles are like ovens that burn calories even when you're at rest. So, more muscle = more calories burned throughout the day. It's like having an automatic calorie-burning mechanism!

It Makes You Feel Good

Have you heard of endorphins? They are those chemicals your body produces during exercise that make you feel amazing. So, in addition to burning calories, exercise puts you in a good mood. It's a two-for-one deal.

Improves Your Overall Health

Beyond weight loss, exercise improves your overall health. It reduces the risk of heart disease, type 2 diabetes, and many other conditions. Additionally, it helps you sleep better, reduces stress, and boosts your energy. In short, it's a miracle drug, but without a prescription!

Fun And Variety

Exercise doesn't have to be boring. In fact, it's usually quite the opposite. There are thousands of ways to move and have fun at the same time. Dancing, swimming, cycling, yoga, playing soccer... or even curling. Whatever makes you happy and gets you moving counts. Find something you enjoy, and it will be easier to maintain the habit.

Socialization

Exercise can be a great way to socialize. Joining a walking group, a sports team, or a fitness class can help you meet new people and stay motivated. And you know, exercising in good company is always more fun.

It's pretty clear, right? Ultimately, physical exercise is crucial for staying fit because, in addition to helping you burn calories, it speeds up your metabolism, improves your health, and makes you feel good. Plus, if you find an activity you enjoy, it can be a lot of fun! So, get off the couch and get moving. Your body - and your mind - will thank you!

Types of Exercise Most Effective for Burning Calories and Improving Health

We've already seen, although we knew it already, that exercise is paramount in our goal of losing weight. So, are you ready to discover how to become a calorie-burning machine while having fun?

Here I present, without complicated jargon, some of the most effective types of exercise to get in shape and improve your health. You choose based on your prior physical fitness, availability, or how motivated you feel that day.

But one thing you always have to be clear about, especially when you come home tired or unmotivated from work: it's better to do 5 minutes of squats in your hallway than spend 5 minutes convincing yourself it's okay not to do them.

Examples of Types of Exercises

Cardio: Sweating Buckets

When the goal is to burn calories, cardio is your best option. Running, swimming, walking, cycling, dancing *Zumba,* or even filming a *TikTok* are excellent choices. These exercises not only make your heart pump faster and stronger but also burn a lot of calories. Think of cardio as that hyperactive friend who always drags you to the dance floor.

Strength Training: Getting Strong Is Cool

Lifting weights, doing push-ups, squats, and other strength exercises help you build muscle. And here's the key: more muscle means more calories burned, even when you're watching your favorite series on the couch. Increased muscle mass requires more energy expenditure, so believe it or not, your metabolism will also increase at rest.

Pro Tip: When you lie down to go to sleep, before starting your usual routines (reading a book, browsing your social media, or simply watching TV before falling asleep), do this: from your supine position (lying on your back, that is) stretch both legs and lift them about 25 in (10 cm) off the surface, in this case, the bed. Keep them raised like this for 30 seconds, rest for another half minute, and repeat this exercise two more times (three times in total is enough to start with). You'll be doing abdominal exercises in a simple way and quickly incorporating them into your routine. Over time, the 30 seconds will increase to a minute and beyond, as much as you want. You'll be burning calories right before falling asleep, sleeping better, and gradually strengthening your abdominal muscles.

HIIT: Burning Calories at Full Speed

Here's the latest in rapid calorie burning: High-Intensity Interval Training (*HIIT*). This exercise is perfect for those with limited time but want great results. Alternate between high-intensity exercises and short rest periods. It's like sprinting and then walking (classic interval training) over and over again. The best part is you can finish a HIIT session in 20-30 minutes and feel like you've trained for hours.

Team Sports: Exercise Disguised As Fun

Playing soccer, basketball, volleyball, or even curling -yes, my healthy obsession with this magnificent ice sport- any team sport is a great way to burn calories without realizing it. You're so focused on the game and having a good time that you forget you're exercising. Plus, don't forget, it's an excellent way to socialize and meet new people. And who knows... maybe we're witnessing a future Olympic promise!

Fitness Classes: Group Energy

Joining a spinning, kickboxing, pilates, or yoga class not only keeps you active but also harnesses the group's energy to motivate you. Fitness classes are ideal if you need a little inspiration and someone to push you to give it your all.

Outdoor Activities: Caloric Adventures

Going for walks, hiking, skating, or even playing frisbee in the park or at the beach are also great ways to exercise outdoors. You get to enjoy the sun, fresh air, and in the process, burn a bunch of calories. It's also a great excuse to explore new places.

Functional Training: Moving Like A Ninja

Functional exercises like burpees, jumps, and mountain climbers enhance your ability to perform daily activities with ease. They help you burn a multitude of calories quickly and strengthen your entire body, preparing you for any challenge life throws your way.

These are just a few specific examples of simple activities you can start right away.

Now it's up to you to assess which type of sport or activity best suits your fitness level. The key takeaway from this list is to apply it to your daily routine. The essence lies in finding the combination of exercises that you enjoy and that keep you moving. Whether you're sweating it out with cardio, getting strong with strength training, or having fun with team sports, there's a world of options to burn calories and improve your health.

Strategies to Incorporate Exercise into Your Daily Routine

But you might be wondering... "I don't even have time for a quick run around the block!"

Do you want to know how to become an exercise pro without juggling your schedule?

Here are some practical and fun strategies to seamlessly incorporate exercise into your daily routine, many of which you can do without leaving the comfort of your home.

Strategies

Get Up And Walk

Starting the day with a bit of exercise can be wonderful. Not an early riser? No problem. Even a couple of stretches or a quick walk around the block can wake up your muscles and get you going.

Make Exercise A Date

Put your daily exercise sessions on your calendar as if they were important meetings. Treat them like non-negotiable appointments, and you'll see how they become part of your routine. Do you have a date with yourself to break a sweat? Absolutely!

Exercise In Small Doses

As I try to explain, you don't have to dedicate a whole hour at the gym if you can't. Divide your exercise into small doses: 10 minutes of walking here, 15 minutes of stretching there, 5 minutes of squats before bedtime. Every bit counts and can be easier to fit into your day.

Make It Social

As we've mentioned, exercising with friends or joining a

fitness class can be excellent motivation. Just the fact of having plans set to meet someone for exercise makes it less likely that you'll back out.

Combine Exercise With Daily Tasks

Take the stairs instead of the elevator; walk or bike to work, if possible; do squats while waiting for the microwave to finish (my obsession with squats is something I need to look into); or do a short session of push-ups before bedtime. Every small movement counts and, as we've mentioned, adds to your daily activity... and to the total calories burned.

Have Fun

Choose activities that you genuinely enjoy. Do you like dancing? Put on some music and dance like nobody's watching! Prefer the outdoors? Try hiking or cycling. Don't want to leave the house? Put on a short exercise video from YouTube and mimic *Jane Fonda* in her prime. If you have fun, it won't feel like an obligation.

Set Achievable Goals

Don't aim to run a marathon on the first day (or the second, speaking from experience). Start with small, achievable goals like walking 10 minutes a day or doing 10 push-ups (I'll skip mentioning squats this time, but they work too).

As you achieve these goals, you'll feel motivated to increase the challenge.

Use Technology

New technologies have come to make our lives easier, and naturally, they can also help us move our bodies and burn calories. There are plenty of apps and devices that can assist you in staying active. From reminders to move, step counters, to fitness challenges, technology can be a great ally in your mission to incorporate exercise into your life.

Find Your Ideal Time

Some people prefer exercising in the morning, others at noon, and some in the evening. Try different times of the day and discover when you feel best exercising. Adjust your routine accordingly. But be cautious, especially in summer, during the peak sun hours. Sweating more doesn't necessarily mean burning more calories (another myth debunked, by the way).

Be Creative

Don't have gym equipment at home? No problem. Use what you have on hand: water bottles as dumbbells, a chair for dips (a type of exercise where you lower and raise your body using your arms on a stable surface), or a towel for stretching exercises. You can also get a pedal roller and turn your regular bike into an impressive stationary bike that lets you pedal while enjoying your favorite TV show. Creativity knows no bounds, and you don't need to spend thousands of euros to have a functional gym setup.

Reward Yourself

And as important as exercising is rewarding yourself after a tough but rewarding session. After finishing, give yourself a small reward. It could be a relaxing bath, an episode of The Simpsons, or a favorite fruit. Rewards keep you motivated and make the effort worthwhile. Just don't deceive yourself and order from Telepizza thinking you've already burned off that family-size pizza. The body doesn't work like that.

As mentioned, the key takeaway from all of this isn't memorizing this or any other list, but using it as a guide to start incorporating exercise into your daily routine without it becoming a headache. With a bit of creativity and some of the tricks already discussed - or others that you can come up with yourself - you can start moving more and enjoying this process.

4. Psychological aspects
in weight loss

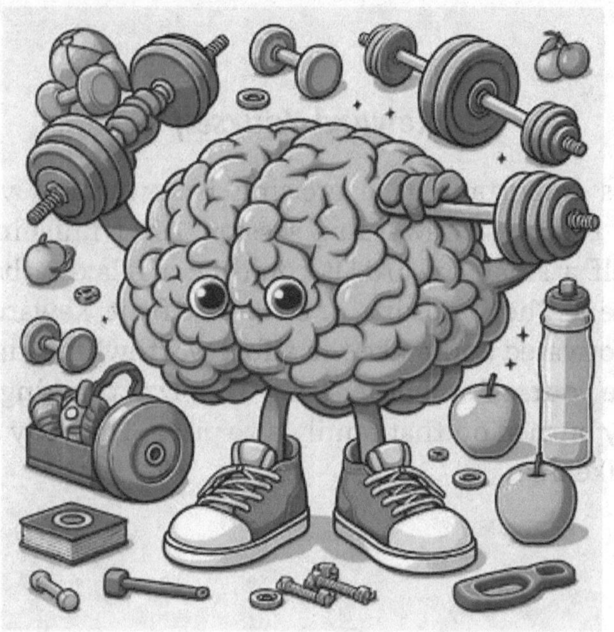

Emotional and Psychological Factors Influencing Body Weight

Did you know that your brain can be a secret conspirator against your battle to achieve a healthy weight? Emotional and psychological factors play a crucial role in how, when, and why we eat.

They are the anti-heroes in our personal struggle, so...

Let's unmask these hidden villains!

The Villains

Emotional Eating: The Carb Hug

Have you ever had a terrible day and all you wanted was a big, chocolatey ice cream? Don't worry, you're not alone. When we're stressed, sad, or bored, it's easy to seek comfort in food. That buttery croissant isn't judging you, but it also doesn't solve your problems. Emotional eating is using food as a temporary patch to mask negative feelings.

Stress: The Silent Saboteur

Stress is a constant companion in our modern lives and can trigger cravings for unhealthy foods. When we're stressed, the body releases cortisol, a hormone that, among many functions, increases appetite. So, when your boss gives you a last-minute task, your brain might whisper, *"Pizza!"*

Anxiety And Depression: The Vicious Cycle

Many people battling anxiety and depression often experience changes in their eating habits. Some eat more, seeking comfort in food, while others lose their appetite altogether. The lack of essential nutrients can worsen these issues, creating a vicious cycle.

Self-Image And Self-Esteem: The Betraying Mirror

Our self-perception, especially negative ones, can influence our eating habits. If you feel insecure or have low self-esteem, you may turn to food for comfort, or conversely, restrict yourself from eating. The key is to work on a positive body image and self-love.

Habits And Environment: The Invisible Influence

Sometimes, we don't even realize how our environment and habits influence our eating. If your friends always want to go out for fast food or if your family has a habit of eating in front of the TV, it's easy to fall into those patterns without thinking. Changing your environment and creating healthy habits can make a big difference. And remember, an occasional beer or wine won't make you gain weight, but four might.

Busy Mind: Mindless Eating

Being constantly busy and distracted can lead to "mindless eating." It's that terrible moment when you realize you've polished off an entire bag of *Ruffles* while engrossed in the finale of *La Casa de Papel*. Being mindful of what you eat and savoring each portion can help you better control your intake.

Good Sleep: The Guardian Of Weight

Contrary to what might seem, lack of sleep can disrupt hormone synthesis that controls hunger, making you feel hungrier and crave high-calorie foods. Getting good sleep not only makes you feel fresher and more rested but also helps keep your weight under control.

W ell, now you're aware that your emotions and mental state have a big impact on your body weight. Recognizing these factors and learning to manage them in a healthy way can help you maintain a balanced weight. So, next time you feel tempted to devour a chocolate bar after a tough day, take a deep breath, go for a walk, or call a friend.

Your brain and your belly will thank you!

Relationship between Food and Emotions

Have you ever felt that a *Kit-Kat* understands you better than anyone? The relationship between food and emotions is a real soap opera, full of ups and downs, dramas, and reconciliations.

Let's take a mental *Kit-Kat* break and explore this relationship.

<u>Food and Emotions</u>

Emotional Eating: The Ups And Downs Of Love

When we're happy, we eat to celebrate; when we're sad, we eat to comfort ourselves. Food becomes our faithful companion, always ready to be there for us. As mentioned, that pizza doesn't judge you if you've had a bad day, and that ice cream doesn't ask why you're crying.

Stress And Its Strange Cravings

Stress is like that buddy who always shows up unannounced and never comes alone. When we're stressed, our body releases the aforementioned cortisol, and suddenly we find ourselves craving all kinds of comforting and unhealthy snacks. It's as if stress says, *"Yes, you need to finish that jar of peanut butter!"*

Anxiety And The Midnight Feast

Anxiety can lead us to the kitchen in search of something to chew on and calm our nerves. Before we know it, we've emptied the fridge, the snack cupboard, and if you push it, the entire pantry. Eating becomes a temporary distraction, a momentary relief from that constant unease.

Sadness And The Carb Hug

When we feel depressed, it's common to seek comfort in carbohydrates. Bread, pasta, and sugar become our best confidants. Why? Because carbohydrates increase serotonin levels in the brain, that chemical that makes us feel good. It's like a warm hug in the form of pastries.

Celebration And Indulgence

On the positive side, we celebrate with food. Birthdays, parties, job promotions, your boss's retirement... any excuse is good to enjoy a hearty and delicious meal, well accompanied by spirits and fermented drinks. Food is part of our celebrations, giving us the opportunity to share happy moments with others.

Boredom And Endless Snacking

Sometimes, often, we eat simply because we're bored. We're sitting at home with nothing to do, and the fridge seems to call out to us. Before we know it, we've gone through all the week's supplies. Sweet or savory, anything goes. It's a form of entertainment that, while not the healthiest, is very common.

Reward And Self-Care

Often, we use food as a reward. *"I've had a tough day, I deserve a burger"*. Or *"I've exercised, I deserve a pastry"*. While indulging occasionally is fine, it's important not to turn food, especially processed food, into our sole source of gratification.

As you can see, the relationship between food and emotions is complex and multifaceted. Our emotions can influence what we eat, when we eat, and how much we eat. Being aware of this relationship allows us to make much healthier decisions and seek other ways to manage our emotions. So, the next time you find yourself on an emotional roller coaster, remember that there are many ways to overcome it, and not all of them come in the form of a hot dog.

Techniques for managing anxiety, stress, and other emotional challenges related to weight loss

Next, we will discuss some techniques that, however simple they may seem, are especially effective in keeping those emotional challenges we've talked about in check, and continuing on your path toward a much healthier lifestyle.

Techniques

Take A Deep Breath And Count To Ten... Or Twenty

When you feel anxiety creeping in, take a deep breath. Inhale through your nose counting to four, hold the breath counting to four, and exhale slowly through your mouth counting again to four (I know, that adds up to twelve, but the more the better). Do this a few times and you'll notice your mind calming down. It's like rebooting your system!

Get Moving!

As we've seen in previous chapters, exercise is an excellent remedy for stress and anxiety. Still, I won't tire of reminding you. Go for a walk, do some burpees (push-ups plus squats), or take the dog for a walk. Movement releases endorphins that will make you feel good and help release tension... and your dog will thank you for it.

Have A Laugh

Laughter truly is the best medicine. Watch an episode of your favorite comedy, look for funny videos on *TikTok*, call that friend who always makes you laugh, or enjoy a funny book. Laughter not only relieves stress but also burns a few calories.

Meditation And Mindfulness: Get Zen!

Meditation and mindfulness can help you be more present and less worried about the future or the past. Dedicate a few minutes each day to sitting quietly, focusing on your breath, and letting your thoughts come and go without judgment. And believe it or not, you also burn calories.

Write Down Your Feelings

Keeping a journal can be very therapeutic. In fact, during this process of changing habits, it's highly recommended. Start todaywrite down how you feel, what worries you, and what makes you happy. Note your achievements and, inevitably, your small setbacks. Gradually, you'll see how successes far outweigh those minor stumbles, which will help you through the toughest moments. Often, getting things out of your mind and onto paper can help you see them from a new perspective.

Listen To Relaxing Music

Music has a powerful effect on our emotions. Create a playlist of your most relaxing songs and listen when you feel stress building up. Close your eyes, relax, and let the music take you to a calmer place.

Connect With Nature

Spending time outdoors can be incredibly relaxing. Take a walk in a park, walk barefoot on grass, or simply sit under a tree. If it's raining, focus on the patter of rain on the window. Nature has a de-stressing effect and helps you disconnect from daily hustle.

Talk To Someone

Sometimes, simply verbalizing how you feel can work wonders. Call a friend, a family member, or even consider talking to a professional if needed. Sharing your concerns and receiving support will lighten your mind (and can help you feel lighter in body too).

Find A Hobby

Keep your mind busy and happy with activities you enjoy. Whether it's painting, cooking (yes, cooking, but watch out for snacking while at it), gardening, or reading a good book. Having a hobby can distract you from stress and anxiety, giving you something positive to focus on.

Practice Gratitude

Every day, take a moment to reflect on everything you're grateful for. It can be as simple as a sunny day, a hot cup of coffee, or a kind smile. And if you're religious, you have another reason to give thanks. Practicing gratitude helps you focus on the positive and reduces anxiety.

Sleep Well

Another point I won't tire of repeating. Sleep is crucial for managing stress and anxiety. Make sure to get enough sleep each night, create a relaxing sleep routine, and try to keep a regular schedule. A good rest can work wonders for your emotional well-being!

So... let's get started!

There you have a series of simple techniques that will help you manage anxiety, stress, and other emotional challenges that hinder your weight loss.

Remember, taking care of your mental health is as important as taking care of your body.

So breathe, relax, and keep moving forward!

5. An integrated approach

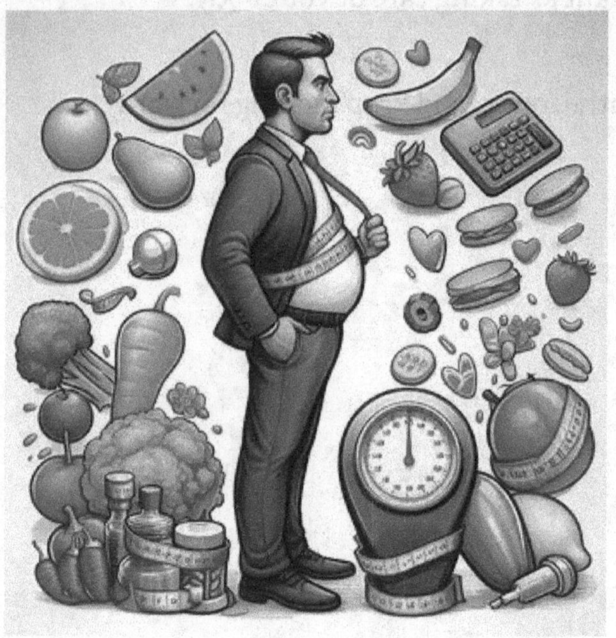

The importance of approaching weight loss from a comprehensive perspective

Throughout these pages, we have been discovering the factors and main aspects that contribute to weight loss... and those that complicate it for us. All of these have been explained separately, but as you will see, they form an integrated perspective that we have been addressing in these pages. An important aspect to consider is that losing weight is not merely achieved by eating less and moving more. Indeed, as mentioned at the beginning of these pages, our ancestors already knew the saying *"less on the plate and more on the shoe"*, but in the society we are immersed in today, that theory falls short, to say the least. If you truly want to see lasting results, you need to adopt a comprehensive perspective.

What does that mean? Let's break it down!

In the first place, it's important to understand that your body and mind are literally inseparable. If you only focus on diet and exercise but neglect your mental health, it's like trying to watch a whole season of *Game of Thrones* skipping half of the episodes. Stress, anxiety, and emotions play a huge role in how you eat and your habits. So, giving your brain a break is as crucial as giving your muscles a rest after a good workout.

It's not just about what you eat, but how you eat. Adopting

healthy eating habits doesn't just mean choosing a salad over a burger (though that helps). It's about enjoying every bite, listening to your body when it says it's full, or avoiding eating in front of the TV. Mindful eating, as we've already explained, can transform your relationship with food and make you enjoy your meals more, even those occasional indulgences that we all deserve.

We've established that exercise shouldn't feel like medieval torture. If you hate running, don't force yourself to do it. If the gym isn't your thing, look for alternatives. Find an activity that brings you joy and embrace it (curling, for example, is a great option; the cold from the ice rink forces your metabolism to burn more calories to maintain body temperature). But seriously (although curling is indeed effective) the key is to stay active in a way that makes you happy. When you enjoy it, you're more likely to stick with the habit. And hey, you might even bring back the *hula-hoop* trend by sharing your sessions on social media.

And yes, back to sleep (hope you didn't doze off!). Don't underestimate the power of a good night's sleep or a short nap (no more than fifteen minutes). Quality sleep regulates the hormonal metabolism that controls hunger and satiety, helping you make better food choices. Plus, you'll feel more energized to tackle your workouts and daily activities. So, consider those sleep hours as part of your weight loss plan. Sweet dreams!

Of course, you don't have to go it alone if you don't want to (neither in sleep nor in exercise). Some people enjoy exercising alone with their music and thoughts, while others prefer the opposite. It's your choice. However, to start off, I always recommend surrounding yourself with supportive people, as this can make a big difference. Whether it's a running buddy, a *WhatsApp* or *Telegram* support group, or simply someone to talk to about your challenges and successes. Any social contact typically provides a safety net to catch you when you falter (because you will) and encourage you to get back up again.

Keep in mind that sustainable weight loss doesn't happen overnight. It's a process that requires time, patience, and sometimes adjusting your expectations. I emphasize the importance of avoiding fad diets and magic shortcuts. Instead, focus on making small, sustainable changes to your lifestyle. Remember, lasting changes are achieved step by step, not in one leap.

Developing a healthy relationship with food is crucial. This means not banning certain foods or labeling them as *"off-limits"*. All foods can fit into a balanced diet if consumed in moderation. The key is learning to enjoy the foods you love without guilt and understanding that an occasional indulgence won't derail your progress. Eating should be a pleasurable experience, not a source of stress. It's just about learning to manage it.

In summary, approaching the goal of achieving a healthy weight from a comprehensive perspective means taking care of your mind, enjoying food, finding physical activities that excite you, sleeping well, seeking support, being patient with yourself, and developing a positive relationship with food. It's not just a physical transformation but a journey toward a healthier and more balanced lifestyle.

And, dear reader, never forget that in certain cases, it's very important to seek advice from a specialized medical professional.

6. Artificial Intelligence in weight loss

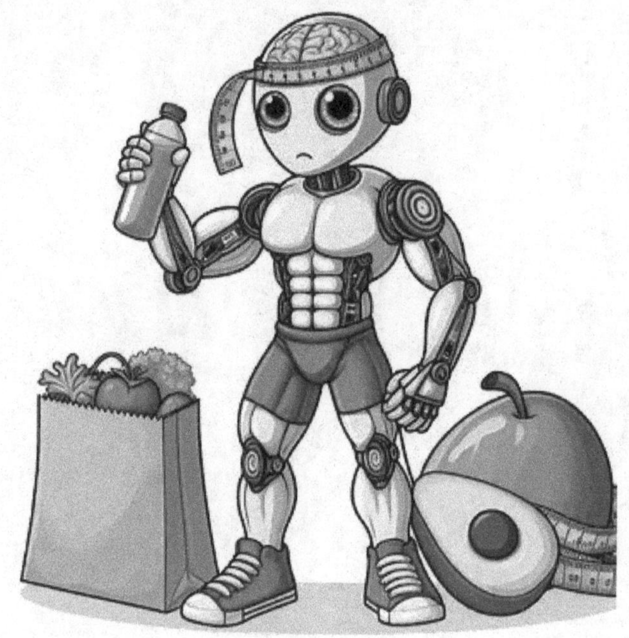

Artificial Intelligence in Weight Loss

Artificial intelligence (AI) is becoming a revolutionary tool in weight management. From customizing diets to creating tailored exercise routines, AI uses data and algorithms to provide precise and effective recommendations.

Imagine having a personal trainer and nutritionist in your pocket, adjusting your plans based on your progress and needs. Furthermore, AI can help identify behavioral and emotional patterns that affect your weight, offering more comprehensive and sustainable solutions.

It is still early to envision the full scope of what is possible, but AI promises to make the weight loss process smarter, personalized, and more accessible.

Applications of Artificial Intelligence in Health and Weight Loss

Imagine having a small personal trainer on your wrist. Yes, we're talking about those super cool wearable devices like smartwatches and fitness bands. These gadgets use artificial intelligence to monitor everything from how many steps you take each day to how many calories you burn while busting your best dance moves in the living room. They can even track your sleep patterns! And all of this without you having to do anything except wear them.

But wait, there's more.

These technologies not only collect data but also provide real-time feedback. *Have you overindulged in pasta?* Your health app will gently let you know. *Need to move more?* Your watch will give you a friendly nudge to get up and take a short walk. It's like having that honest friend nearby who always tells you the truth, but in a digital version.

And let's not forget mobile applications. These apps, which we are already so accustomed to, use AI to analyze your behavioral patterns and offer personalized recommendations. For example, if you tend to eat more when stressed, your app can suggest relaxation techniques or remind you to drink more water. Additionally, you can track your food intake, exercises, and even your mood.

Best of all, these technologies keep you motivated. Want to achieve a goal? Set targets in your app and celebrate each milestone with medals or other virtual rewards. In many cases, it can feel like playing a real video game where you are the main character.

Furthermore, future AI could create hyper-personalized weight loss plans based on your genes, microbiota, and other scientific factors. Generic diets will be a thing of the past; every bite you take will be specifically designed for your body and its needs.

And let's not forget augmented reality (AR). Imagine wearing AR glasses and seeing your meals transform into healthy options before your eyes. You could even exercise in virtual worlds, running on the beach or climbing mountains without leaving your own room.

Another incredible trend will be devices that integrate even more into your daily life. Think of smart clothing that monitors your health, shoes that track your physical activity, and even plates that count the calories in your food. AI will be everywhere, ensuring that you're always in your best shape.

Amidst all this technological whirlwind, accessibility will be key. Advanced technologies will be within everyone's reach, not just gadget enthusiasts. From free apps to affordable devices, everyone will be able to benefit from these innovations regardless of their budget.

With all that said, I want to clarify that it's not my intention to advertise any specific app, as each has its own unique features. You just need to go to the *Play Store* or *App Store* (depending on whether you use *Android* or *Apple*) and explore the multitude of apps for sports activities and/or weight loss that you'll find there. Perhaps in a follow-up, I'll provide a detailed analysis of the apps that I believe are most useful and effective, as well as expand on this extensive and exciting topic. But for now, all you need to know is that these tools exist and they can help you a lot in achieving the goal we've set.

In conclusion, wearable devices and mobile apps are making health tracking fun, accessible, and super efficient. With the help of AI, you can monitor your progress and receive useful tips in real-time, ensuring you're always on the right path towards your health and wellness goals starting right now.

Give technology a chance and let it help you achieve your goals in an easy and enjoyable way!

7. And now... Let´s get started!

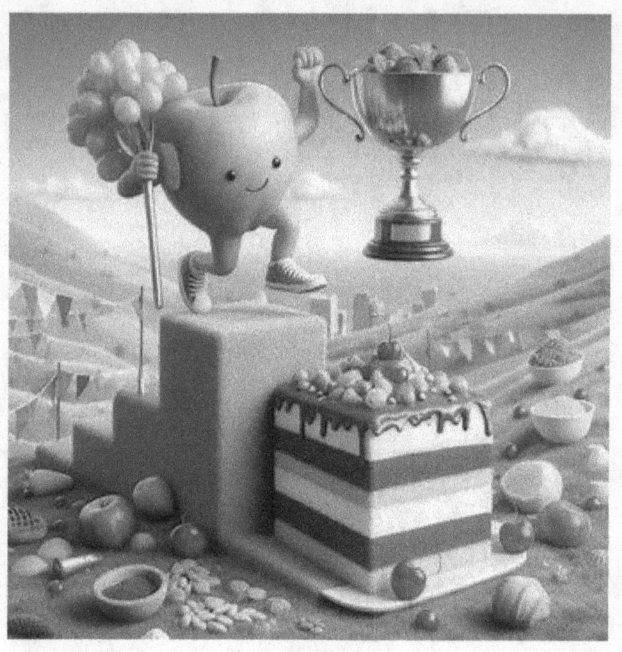

And now... let's begin!

Finally, it's time to recap everything we've learned and, without excuses, get started on our goal: achieving a healthy and satisfying weight.

Firstly, just for having trusted this work to address your weight loss project, I provide you with my professional email in case you still have any questions. I'll be happy to try to help you resolve them:

benemeritodoctor@gmail.com

<u>Conclusions</u>

Now, let's summarize the main stages we face in our project, which I insist must begin today, to achieve a healthy and fit weight.

The problem of obesity and overweight

We started this long race with a big question: why is obesity such an important issue today? And we've seen how this epidemic has grown in our society like a *Gremlin* swimming in a pool.

Multiple perspectives

It's clear to us that there's no magic solution. Simply wishing to lose weight isn't enough! We need to approach it from all angles: nutrition, exercise, mental health, and even social and genetic factors. It's like a great recipe that needs all its ingredients to work.

Foundations of Healthy Eating

We've debunked the myth that eating healthy is boring. Here's where we've learned that a balanced diet can include a bit of everything, from proteins to, occasionally, your favorite snacks, as long as you keep it balanced. Yes, there's even room for chocolate!

Myths and truths about diets

We also learned not to trust most of the myths circulating on social media and among our acquaintances about diets. Just celery for meals? No, thank you! We've discovered that many *"quick fixes"* are nothing more than fairy tales and that sustainable paths are much more effective.

Practical tips for improving your diet

We discussed how small changes can make a big difference. Make the nutritional decalogue your own, and you'll see results from day one. And don't forget the importance of enjoying every bite!

The Value of Physical Exercise

There's no doubt about the importance of exercise, but it doesn't have to feel like a punishment. It can and should be fun and varied. Dancing in your kitchen while cooking, taking a walk with friends, or doing a round of burpees down the hallway; the important thing is to keep moving.

Types of Exercise

We've explored and analyzed various calorie-burning exercises like they're paper in a barbecue. Cardio, strength training, yoga, abs... You know it... It all counts!

Strategies for Incorporating Exercise

We've also learned various tricks to make exercise a natural part of our daily routine. Goodbye, laziness! Incorporating movement can be as simple as taking the stairs instead of the elevator.

Emotional and Psychological Factors

We've shed light on our minds. We now know that our emotions play a huge role in our weight. Emotional eating is real, and learning to manage our emotions is key to success.

Relationship Between Food and Emotions

We've seen how often we eat not because we're hungry, but because we're bored, sad, or stressed. It's time to break those patterns!

Techniques for Managing Anxiety and Stress

We've discussed techniques like meditation, mindfulness,

or simply taking a moment to breathe deeply. Mental peace is as important as physical peace.

Comprehensive Approach to Weight Loss

We've also seen that, to succeed in weight loss, we need a comprehensive approach. It's not just about what we eat or how much we move, but also about how we feel and think.

Integration of Nutrition, Exercise, and Mental Health

We've learned to combine all of this into a unique and personalized plan. The synergy between nutrition, exercise, and mental health is the secret recipe for lasting change.

AI in Weight Loss

And last but not least, we've explored how artificial intelligence is changing the game. From mobile applications to wearable devices, technology is here to make our lives easier and our weight loss more effective.

But now that I know all the theory... how do I put it into practice?

Well, you're right.

Now that we understand all the factors that will influence and help us achieve our healthy weight, we need to know how and when to implement the plan.

So, grab your calendar, mark today as the start of your new life, and begin gaining in health.

Put it into practice

Visualize your goal

Imagine how you will feel when you achieve your objective. Not just physically, but mentally as well. Set a realistic goal and envision that sense of accomplishment, that extra confidence, and that overflowing energy. To reach the goal, you need to start with the starting gun.

Small steps, big achievements

Remember, you don't have to change everything overnight. Start today with small changes, like drinking more water, having those two glasses before every meal (one during dinners), or taking the stairs instead of the elevator. Each small step after you start today brings you closer to your goal, and before you know it, those steps will add up to a great transformation.

Find your fun exercise

Exercise doesn't have to be torture. If you already have an exercise you enjoy, jot it down. If you haven't decided yet, search for *"fun home exercises"* online, and you're sure to find something you truly enjoy. If you have fun, it won't feel like work but rather a hobby you look forward to. Remember, as the saying goes, if you do what you love, you'll never work a day in your life.

Celebrate every victory

Don't wait until the end to celebrate. Every time you reach a milestone, no matter how small, celebrate it! Whether it's losing a kilo, completing a week of workouts, maintaining your streak in the app, or simply feeling more energetic. Every victory is a step forward.

Surround yourself with support

Start looking for friends, family, or an online community to support and motivate you. Share your achievements and challenges with them, either through the app itself or with a post on Instagram or Facebook. A good support system can work wonders in any project.

Be kind to yourself

There will be good days and bad days, and that's okay. Don't punish yourself for setbacks; instead, see them as opportunities to learn and grow. Self-compassion is key to maintaining long-term motivation.

Make it yours

Remember, this is your journey. What works for others may not necessarily work for you. Customize your plan according to your preferences and needs. This will not only make it more effective but also more sustainable.

Draw inspiration from real stories

Read real-life stories of people who have achieved their weight loss goals. Seeing how others have overcome similar challenges can give you the extra push you need to keep going. Perhaps you will become the prototype that others look up to later on.

Lean on professionals

Sometimes, in addition to our willpower and an efficient plan, the help of professionals is necessary. If your weight loss needs to exceed 15% of your current weight, it's advisable to discuss this with your doctor. They may be able to assist with medication or refer you to another specialist to facilitate your journey.

Great, we're ready and motivated to the max! The journey starts right now. Don't stress out, and remember that if many people have achieved it, you can too.

And now that you know why you weren't losing weight, you'll only be left to reconsider the question...

Why wasn't I losing weight?

About the Author

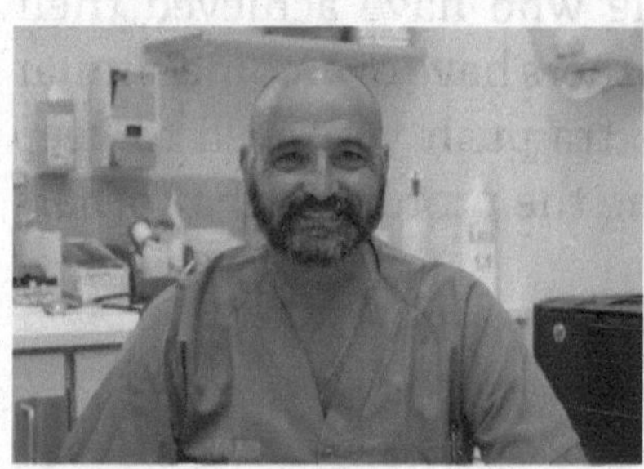

Born in Zaragoza (Spain) in 1975, he joined the Spanish Army in the nineties and later transferred to the Guardia Civil (Spanish Police) where he served for nearly fourteen years in various positions, including the elite GRS (Group of Reserve and Security) unit of the Guardia Civil. During his tenure as a distinguished agent, he pursued studies in Education and later in Medicine, both at the University of Zaragoza.

As a physician, he specialized in Radiation Oncology and obtained postgraduate degrees in Clinical Dermatology from the Catholic University of Valencia and in Aesthetic Medicine and Anti-Aging from the Complutense University of Madrid.

He has authored several books, including the entertaining *Benemérito Doctor* series, presented various medical lectures, and conducted several scientific studies. Currently, he practices as a Hospital Emergency Physician and as an Aesthetic Medicine Specialist.

Important

This book is a *beta* version, which means its intention is to improve over time based on the needs of the readers. Your feedback is essential for this process.

Please leave a review on Amazon and let me know what you thought.

What did you like the most? Is there anything you missed? Would you add or remove any parts?

Thank you very much!

Other Books By This Author

You can access other books by the author through their author page on Amazon.

9 798339 050575